The Salt Counter

compiled by Michael Wright
with a foreword by
Dr Alan Maryon Davis

The
Salt Counter

Pan Original Pan Books

First published 1984 by Pan Books Ltd,
Cavaye Place, London SW10 9PG
© Michael Wright 1984
ISBN 0 330 26934 8
Photoset by Parket Typesetting Service, Leicester
Printed in Great Britain by
Hunt Barnard Printing Ltd, Aylesbury

Contents

Foreword

Dr Alan Maryon Davis MB BChir MSc MRCP MFCM
Medical Officer to the Health Education Council

Did you know that every year you scoff about half a ton of food and quaff about 200 gallons of drink? So it's hardly surprising that you are what you eat, and that your day-to-day diet can have a profound effect on your health as well as your waistline.

A few decades ago good nutrition meant getting enough energy, protein, vitamins and minerals for healthy growth and repair of the body's tissues. Today the biggest nutritional problem in this country is that too many people are eating too much of the sorts of foods that can all too easily lead to chronic ill-health. Too much fatty food, too much sugar and other refined carbohydrates can all contribute to obesity and other related problems such as diabetes and coronary heart disease.

Now another everyday item in our diet has come under suspicion as a potential source of danger. Salt. Common salt, otherwise known as sodium chloride. Or to be more precise, the sodium part of it. As more and more research results come in, the case against sodium is getting stronger and stronger, and many national advisory bodies on nutrition and health are now advocating a reduced salt intake. In Britain, the Health Education Council recommends that the average person should cut down their everyday salt intake by about 25 per cent. To do so, says the HEC, 'could be very good for you. It certainly won't do you any harm'. So how can you start to cut down?

The best thing is to do it in easy stages, starting with the salt cellar on the table. Shake less and less on your food. Then use less and less in cooking. As every good cook knows, a little seasoning goes a long way, and you'll be surprised how soon you get used to the more subtle flavours in your favourite dishes. But the way to really make an impact on your overall sodium intake is to keep a close eye on what you buy. There's no doubt that by checking the sodium content of what goes into your shopping basket, you can achieve the biggest reductions. The snag is that hardly any food products have their sodium content marked on the label. That's why I think this book is so useful. It provides a comprehensive list of everyday foods with their sodium content at a glance.

So, if you care about what that annual half-ton of food and 200 gallons of drink might be doing to your health, I recommend you take this handy guide with you on your next saunter round the supermarket shelves.

You never know, it could change your life.

Alan Maryon Davis
July 1983

Introduction

We take salt so much for granted as a food flavouring that we forget that in ancient times it was a valued commodity to be traded over vast distances, used as a currency, taxed, and even fought over. As a result, it has entered our language in ways far removed from its current mundane status. People may be 'the salt of the earth' or 'worth their salt', collecting their pay cheque every month little suspecting that the word *salary* comes from the Latin for *salt money*.

Today, we take our food with rather more than the proverbial 'pinch of salt', each consuming on average 4.5kg, or 10lbs, of salt every year – about 12 grams or 2½ teaspoonsful each day. Apart from sprinkling it from the salt-cellar and spooning it into the cooking pot, much salt is used in preserved and processed foods as well as occurring naturally in greater or lesser amounts in just about everything we eat.

But, as with many things we take for granted, hidden dangers have recently become apparent in this commonest of all food additives. Eating too much salt, it seems, can be bad for your health. Correction; eating too much *sodium* can be bad for your health. Sodium (whose chemical symbol is Na) is, as you may recall from school chemistry lessons, one of the two chemical elements making up common salt. The other is chlorine (Cl). Chemically speaking, salt is sodium chloride (NaCl), sodium accounting for about 40 per cent and chlorine about 60 per cent of salt's weight.

The culprit, it seems, is the sodium, and this means that

many other food additives and ingredients containing sodium add to the medical hazard of consuming too much salt. Salt is the main source of sodium in most people's diet, but baking soda (and baking powder) come a close second. Other sources include preservatives such as sodium benzoate, sodium nitrite and sodium sulphite, the flavour-enhancer monosodium glutamate (usually known simply as MSG), and such additives as sodium polyphosphates (used to help bind flakes of fish into fish fingers) and even vitamin C (often added in the form of sodium ascorbate).

No one is suggesting that these should be banished from your plate at a stroke. Indeed, sodium is an essential part of everyone's diet. Possibly a relic of the time when our ancient ancestors crawled from the salty seas millions of years ago, all our body tissues are bathed in a kind of weak brine, and our bloodstream itself is salty. In fact, the correct salt balance is vital for the proper functioning of the body – in particular, the transmission of signals along nerves and the beating of the heart depend on it. The job of maintaining this balance is mainly the kidneys'; any excess sodium is excreted in the urine and, to a lesser extent, sweat.

The remarkable thing is how little sodium the body needs in relation to most people's intake. It is believed that most adults can remain healthy on less than half a gram of salt (or, to be precise, 200 milligrams of sodium) a day – less than 5 per cent of their average consumption. The other 95 per cent is promptly got rid of. (Needs do rise in special circumstances, such as heavy manual labour or other exertion in high temperatures, or diarrhoea causing loss of body fluids, but here I am talking about the average person working in a normal environment.)

There, it seems, for very many people the story ends. Salt and other forms of sodium surplus to the body's needs are efficiently excreted and they are no worse for it. But for others, for reasons that are not fully understood, the result may be raised blood pressure (or hypertension) and, with it, a greater risk of heart disease and stroke (brain haemorrhage).

The evidence for the link, as with the link between smoking and lung cancer, is largely circumstantial, but it has been borne out by a number of health studies over recent years. It seems no coincidence, for example, that the country whose population has the highest blood pressures in the world – where stroke is the leading cause of death – should be that with probably the highest salt consumption: Japan, where people's diet is rich in such items as fish, seaweed, salted and pickled vegetables, and soy sauce. Again, in the Solomon Islands, researchers found significantly higher blood pressure among people whose diet contains a lot of salty foods than among otherwise very similar tribes consuming little salt.

The evidence is not always so clear-cut, but most medical workers in this field now feel that there is a clear link between excessive sodium consumption and high blood pressure – though probably only for a proportion of people. It seems that some people have an inborn, inherited proneness to hypertension; these people, if they consume too much sodium, are likely to develop high blood pressure. Others, without the inborn predisposition, can get away with it. The problem is that – apart from looking at family history, for hypertension does tend to run in families – no one can yet tell who is likely to become hypertensive until it happens. (And even then it is very likely to go undetected, perhaps for many years, unless discovered during a routine medical examination.)

In Britain, the number of people who actually have high blood pressure – many of them at only a mild level – has been estimated by the Royal College of General Practitioners at 13 per cent of the adult population – about one in eight. Another calculation suggests that a quarter of the over-45s are hypertensive. But it has been suggested that as many as 40 per cent of people may be susceptible, with black people being significantly more at risk than white, for reasons that can only be guessed at.

So there is ample reason to be careful about how much salt you eat. Official British advice is so far a lot more muted than in America, where nearly half the population are trying to reduce their salt intake. While a low-salt diet is more or less a standard part of the treatment for serious hypertension, the British Nutrition Foundation in a recent working paper suggested that 'at present the evidence relating salt intake to hypertension is not strong enough to recommend a reduction of dietary salt intake for the whole population, but only for susceptible individuals'. But it then goes on to concede that 'a reduction in the average salt intake of the whole population would have no adverse physiological effects, except for the small number who have to do heavy work in hot conditions, *and might have benefits*' (my italics).

Dr Allan Forbes of the US Food and Drug Administration is much more positive: 'Many medical experts believe it is reasonable to modify the sodium intake for everyone.' And that is one of the most cautious statements in a country where no-salt and low-salt eating has become something approaching a hysterical craze and TV commercials for salt-substitutes ask, 'Are you a saltaholic?'

The Health Education Council has gone as far as any official body in Britain so far in condemning salt. It says, 'At the very least, the case against salt is strong enough to suggest that it might be wise for us to cut down on it . . . [Cutting down] could be very good for you. *It certainly won't do you any harm.*' It then goes on to suggest a level of about 9 grams a day, a reduction of 25 per cent from average consumption – still far above the minimum the body needs and a level (9 grams, that is) which the British Nutrition Foundation admits contains 'a very large safety margin'.

The truth is that, as you will see from the tables of sodium content in this book, many of the foods that make up most people's everyday diet contain large amounts of sodium, and there is little risk of anyone other than the raw fruit and vegetable fanatic coming anywhere near the minimum level. (Remember that 12 grams of salt is equivalent to only 4.8 grams – or 4,800 milligrams – of sodium.) To take just one example, a mere 1½ ounces of Cheddar or Cheshire cheese will take you over the bare minimum daily level.

I cannot here recommend a specific figure for you to aim at, but the American Heart Association has issued guidelines for three levels of sodium-restricted diet. 'Mild' restriction corresponds to 2 to 3 grams of sodium (equivalent to 5 to 7.5 grams of salt) per day. A level of 1 gram (1,000 milligrams) of sodium (equal to 2.5 grams of salt) represents 'moderate' restriction, and is often advised for people with severe hypertension. 'Strict' restriction – corresponding to 500 milligrams of sodium, or 1,250 milligrams of salt – is used for patients with heart failure and certain other conditions.

The problem is, of course, that the less salt is used, the less palatable food becomes – a major reason, along with its preservative powers, why food manufacturers salt so many of their products. The 'strict' diet is distinctly unpalatable and bland, but the AHA notes that adjusting to the 'mild'-restriction diet is quite easy. This (corresponding to a halving of average sodium intake) represents a reasonable target for anyone wanting to reduce the risk of hypertension – *subject to any advice your doctor may give you*. If you have any chronic medical condition, particularly of the heart, circulation or kidneys, you should take medical advice before embarking on any major change in your diet. And the same applies, of course, if you suspect that you already have high blood pressure – in which case, you *may* be advised to cut your sodium consumption to the 'moderately' restricted level.

The aim of this guide is to help you find out how much sodium you are consuming and to identify the foods you should cut out or cut down on in order to reduce that figure. Obvious taboo foods are things like bacon, olives, shellfish, salted peanuts and the like. When you think about it, it is not surprising that pickles, most cheese and a lot of other savoury foods are also high in sodium, but you may be more surprised to see the high sodium content of most (but not all) breakfast cereals and bakery products. Another general lesson to be learned is that canned vegetables, soups, meats and so on are generally high in sodium – in the case of most vegetables much more so than their frozen equivalents. You may want to add salt in the cooking of frozen vegetables, but at least the quantity you use is within your control. Hints on palatable low-sodium cooking are given on page 81–6.

As part of any programme to reduce your sodium intake you should get into the habit of reading the ingredient lists on food labels. Steer clear particularly of foods where salt or other sodium compounds appear high up in the list of ingredients. Sometimes the sodium may be 'disguised'; on page 16 I have listed some danger words to look out for. Nor are foods and drinks the only sources of sodium in your diet; as you will see on page 88, a number of over-the-counter medicines are also high in sodium, particularly effervescent indigestion powders and suchlike.

But the point at which to start your salt-reduction campaign is in your own home: with the salt-cellar and the cooking-salt jar. Studies have shown that 'discretionary' use of salt accounts for 25 to 30 per cent of daily intake; most people could make significant reductions here. Australian researchers recently suggested that the way to reduce salt consumption is to make the holes in salt-cellars smaller. Most people, it seems, reach for the salt automatically and without bothering to test their food to see whether it *needs* any extra. With smaller holes, that automatic shake does less harm.

Perhaps the salt-cellar would be better locked away altogether; certainly you should make a conscious effort to use less salt in cooking and on your plate. With the help of this book you can combine such self-restraint with an awareness of foods that will help or hinder your efforts. You can take heart from one common finding of people who cut down on their salt intake: Although food may seem bland at first, the taste buds soon adjust. Not only will you begin to appreciate more the natural flavours of your food, but your sensitivity to salt will increase, and the heavily-salted food you are used to at the moment will probably seem revoltingly briny.

Note

The tables that follow list the sodium content (in milligrams per 100 grams and miligrams per ounce – or, in the case of drinks, per 100 millilitres and per fluid ounce) for more than 1,200 common foods, both fresh and processed. Unless otherwise stated, they are for the food in its fresh, uncooked state, and apply to the edible parts only – that is, excluding bones, shells, etc. Cooking will alter sodium content to a greater or lesser extent: steaming or boiling without salt will reduce the level; cooking with salt will increase it; grilling or frying will have little effect unless salt is added. In the case of canned vegetables, the figures apply to the drained portion – that is, the vegetables themselves without the fluid they float in – but for baked beans and canned fruits, where the whole contents are eaten, the figures apply to the total edible part.

A number of common made-up dishes are included, based on typical standard recipes, but the sodium content of these will of course vary, depending on the amount of salt, baking powder and so on that you use. In general, the figures for dry mixes and dehydrated foods are given for the product in the dry state; diluting them or mixing them with water will of course reduce the effective sodium content per 100 grams, often very considerably – again, the exact final figure will depend on how much water you add.

In the case of most unbranded foods, the figures given are taken from McCance and Widdowson's *The Composition of Foods* (4th edition by A. A. Paul and D. A. T. Southgate of the Medical Research Council, published by Her Majesty's Stationery Office in 1978). These, even when referring to manufactured foods, represent average figures, and will vary from season to season and from manufacturer to manufacturer. In some cases, British figures are not available and published American data have been taken; this is indicated in the tables.

I have also been fortunate in receiving the cooperation of a large number of food manufacturers who have given me figures for the sodium content of their foods – generally obtained by chemical analysis, but in some cases by calculation from the lists of ingredients used, a less accurate method. In any case, these figures too may vary a little with the seasons and of course apply only to the specified brands, but they are a good indication and I am very grateful to the food scientists, analysts and quality control managers concerned for supplying them.

Danger signals

As well as the words *sodium* and *soda* in any context, all the following in an ingredient list usually signal sodium:

Baking powder
Baking soda
Bicarbonate of soda
Brine or brined
Cured
Disodium (eg, disodium
  phosphate)
Kippered

Monosodium (eg,
  monosodium glutamate)
MSG
Na
Salt or salted
Self-raising
Smoked

Abbreviations and some conversion factors

1 gram (g) = 1,000 milligrams (mg)
1 ounce (oz) = 28g
100g = 3½oz
100 millilitres (ml) = 3½ fluid ounces (fl oz)
1 average teacup (5 fl oz) = 140ml, approximately
1 pint = 20 fl oz = 565ml

Food listings

Product	Brand/comments	Na (mg/100g)	Na (mg/oz)
Ackee (canned)		240	68
All-Bran	Kellogg's	1,530	433
Almonds (shelled)		6	1.7
Almonds (shelled, roasted and salted)	(US figs)	200	57
Alpen	Weetabix	170	48
Anchovies (canned in oil)	no exact figures but very high		
Anchovy paste	(US figs)	12,100	3,430
Apple (dried)	(US figs)	4–88	1–25
Apple (fresh)		2	0.6
Apple crumble	(home-made)	68	19
Apple pie	Mr Kipling	92	26
Apple sauce: see under Sauce			
Apricots (canned)		1	0.3
Apricots (dried; raw)		56	16
Apricots (dried; stewed)		20	6
Apricots (fresh; raws or stewed)		trace	trace
Arrowroot		5	1.4
Artichoke, globe (boiled)		15	4.2
Artichokes, Jerusalem		3	0.8
Asparagus (canned)	(US figs)	200–400	57–113
Asparagus (fresh)		2	0.6
Aubergine		3	0.8
Avocado (weighed without stone)		2	0.6

Product	Brand/comments	Na (mg/100g)	Na (mg/oz)
Bacon, generally (lean)		1,870	530
Bacon, generally (fat)		560	159
Bacon, back		1,470	416
Bacon, back	Pork Farms	1,200	340
Bacon, collar		1,690	479
Bacon, gammon		1,180	334
Bacon, streaky		1,500	425
Bacon, streaky	Pork Farms	900	255
Bacon, sweetcure (lean)		1,200	340
Bakewell tarts	Mr Kipling	143	40
Baking powder, regular		11,800	3.34
Baking powder, sodium-free		trace	trace
Baking soda		27,400	7,760
Bananas		1	0.3
Barley, pearl (raw)		3	0.8
Barcelona nuts (shelled)		3	0.8
Beans, baked (canned)	(average)	480	136
Beans, baked (canned)	Hartley's	473	134
Beans, baked (canned)	Heinz	560	159
Beans, baked, with pork sausages (canned)	Heinz	680	193
Beans, broad (canned)	Hartley's	270	76
Beans, broad (fresh; boiled)		20	5.7
Beans, broad (frozen)	Findus	3	0.8
Beans, butter (canned)	Del Monte	276	78
Beans, butter (dried)		62	18
Beans, curried, with sultanas (canned)	Heinz	450	127

Product	Brand/comments	Na (mg/100g)	Na (mg/oz)
Beans, French (canned)	Del Monte	392	111
Beans, French (fresh)		3	0.8
Beans, French (frozen)	Findus	5	1.4
Beans, haricot (dried)		43	12
Beans, mung		28	8
Beans, red kidney (dried)		40	11
Beans, runner (fresh or frozen)		2	0.6
Bean sprouts (canned)	(average)	80	23
Beef (fresh, generally)			
Beef (lean)		61	17
Beef (fat)		33	9.4
Beef, roasted in gravy	Findus	340	96
Beef (salted, dried)	(US figs)	3,900–4,400	1,105–240
Beef, salt silverside (lean and fat)		910	258
Beef, salt silverside (lean only)		1,000	283
Beef and onion pie filling	Tyne Brand	500–600	142–70
Beefburger (fresh, unsalted)		same as beef	
Beefburger (frozen)	(average)	600	170
Beefburgers, Original (frozen)	Birds Eye	430	122
Beefburgers, 100% (frozen)	Birds Eye	260	74
Beefburgers, All Beef (frozen)	Findus	600	170
Beefburgers, 90% (frozen)	Findus	600	170
Beef pie (frozen)	Findus	733	208
Beef pie filling (braised)	Tyne Brand	670	190
Beet, leaf	(US figs)	130	37

Product	Brand/comments	Na (mg/100g)	Na (mg/oz)
Beetroot (raw)		84	24
Bemax	Beechams	4	1.1
Bicarbonate of soda		27,380	7,756
Bilberries (fresh or frozen)		1	0.3
Biscuits: Bath Oliver	Fortts	610	173
Bourbon		50–70	14–20
Cheese: see under Crackers			
Chocolate (full-coated)		160	45
Chocolate Chip	Huntley & Palmer	304	86
Chocolate Digestive, milk		450–90	128–39
Chocolate Digestive, Plain		445–575	126–63
Club	Jacob's	107–96	30–56
Cornish Wafer	Jacob's	476	135
Cream Crackers: see under Crackers			
Custard Cream	Crawford's	142	40
Custard Cream	Peak Frean	117	33
Digestive (plain)		440–615	125–74
Fig Roll	Jacob's	281	80
Fruit Shortcake	McVitie's	227	64
Garibaldi	Peak Frean	172	49
Ginger Nut	(average)	330	94
Ginger Nut	McVitie's	405	115
Ginger Nut	Peak Frean	261	74
Gluten-free	Farley's	57	16
Lincoln	Peak Frean	337	95
Low-Protein	Aproten	30	8.5
Low-Protein	Rite-Diet	10–20	2.8–5.7
Matzo	Rakusen	17	4.8

Product	Brand/comments	Na (mg/100g)	Na (mg/oz)
Nice	Peak Frean	258	73
Oatcake		1,230	348
Rich tea	(average)	410	116
Sandwich		220	62
Shortcake	(average)	360	102
Shortcake	Peak Frean	301	85
Wafer (filled)		70	20
Water		470	133
Water	Jacob's	417	118
see also Crackers, Rusks, Shortbread, brand names			
Blackberries (fresh)		4	1.1
Blackberries (canned)		4	1.1
Blackcurrants		3	0.8
Black pudding (fried)	(average)	1,210	343
Blancmange	(US figs)	65	18
Bloaters (grilled)		700	198
Bouillon cubes: see stock cubes			
Bounty Bar	Mars Ltd	140–45	40–41
Bovril (undiluted)		4,800	1,360
Brains (calf or lamb)		140	40
Bran, Farmhouse	Weetabix	620	176
Bran, wheat (natural)		28	7.9
Bran Buds	Kellogg's	940	266
Bran Fare	Weetabix	50	14
Bran Flakes	Kellogg's	940	266
Bran Flakes	Nabisco	941	267
Brawn	(average)	750	212
Brazil nuts (shelled)		2	0.6
Brazil nuts (shelled, roasted and salted)	(US figs)	190	54
Bread, brown	(average)	550	156

Product	Brand/comments	Na (mg/100g)	Na (mg/oz)
Bread, brown	Hovis	590	167
Bread, currant		160	45
Bread, Granary	Windmill	560	159
Bread, low-sodium (canned)	Rite-Diet	10	2.8
Bread, malt		280	79
Bread, pumpernickel	(US figs)	650–725	184–205
Bread, soda		410	116
Bread, white		540–610	153–73
Bread, wholemeal		540–80	153–64
Bread-and-butter pudding	(home-made)	150	42
Breadcrumbs, white (dried)		760	215
Broccoli spears (fresh or frozen)		12	3.4
Brussels sprouts (fresh or frozen)		4	1.1
Buns, currant	(average)	100	28
Buns, currant (Spicy)	Mother's Pride	210	59
Butter, salted	(average)	870	246
Butter, unsalted		7	2
Butterscotch	Callard & Bowser's	700	198

Product	Brand/comments	Na (mg/100g)	Na (mg/oz)
Cabbage, red (fresh)		32	9.1
Cabbage, red (pickled)	Haywards	850	241
Cabbage, savoy (fresh)		23	6.5
Cabbage, spring (fresh)		12	3.4
Cabbage, white (fresh)		7	2
Cabbage, winter (fresh)		7	2
Cakes: Arctic Gateau (frozen)	Birds Eye	100	28
Arctic Log (frozen)	Birds Eye	140	40
Cherry Fruit	McVitie's	190	54
Cherry Fruit	Mr Kipling	291	82
Chocolate Fudge	Mr Kipling	339	96
Fancy iced	(average)	250	71
Fruit (plain)	(average)	250	71
Fruit (rich)	(home-made)	170	48
Fruit (rich, iced)	(home-made)	120	34
Ginger	McVitie's	456	129
Ginger	Mr Kipling	524	148
Gingerbread	(home-made)	380	108
Madeira	(average)	380	108
Madeira	Mr Kipling	344	97
Rock		480	136
Sponge (no fat; whisking method)	(home-made)	82	23
Sponge (with fat; creaming method)	(home-made)	350	99
Swiss roll (jam)	(average)	420	119
Swiss roll (chocolate)	Cadbury's	203	58
Swiss roll (jam)	Mr Kipling	298	84
Victoria sponge		350	99
Canneloni (frozen)	Findus	404	114

Product	Brand/comments	Na (mg/100g)	Na (mg/oz)
Capers (pickled)	(US figs)	1,800	510
Caramac	Rowntrees	100	28
Caraway seeds	(US figs)	46	13
Cardamom		trace	trace
Carp	(US figs)	15	4.2
Carrots (canned)	(average)	280	79
Carrots (canned, sliced)	Hartley's	481	136
Carrots (canned, whole)	Hartley's	306	87
Carrots (canned)	Del Monte	206	58
Carrots (dried)	(US figs)	268	76
Carrots (fresh – old)		95	27
Carrots (fresh – young)		23	6.5
Cashew nuts (roasted and salted)	KP	380–580	108–64
Cashew nuts (unsalted)		14	4
Casilan	Farley/Glaxo	7	2
Casserole mixes – various flavours (dry weight)	Colman's	5,400–8,600	1,530–2,436
Cauliflower (fresh or frozen)		8	2.3
Caviar	(US figs)	2,200	623
Caviar substitute (lumpfish roe)	Marina	2,750	779
Celeriac (boiled)		28	7.9
Celery		140	40
Celery leaves (fresh)	(US figs)	96	27
Celery salt	Schwartz	29,115	8,250
Celery seed		140	40
Chapatis (made with fat)		130	37
Chapatis (without fat)		120	34
Cheese: Caerphilly	St Ivel	410	116

Product	Brand/comments	Na (mg/100g)	Na (mg/oz)
Camembert		1,410	399
Cheddar	Eden Vale	847	240
Cheddar	St Ivel	660	187
Cheshire	Eden Vale	550	156
Cheshire	St Ivel	530	150
Cottage		410–50	116–27
Cottage (flavoured)		310–530	88–150
Cream		300	85
Danish Blue		1,420	402
Derbyshire	St Ivel	570	161
Double Gloucester	St Ivel	570	161
Edam		980	278
Gorgonzola	(US figs)	1,400	397
Lancashire	St Ivel	590	167
Leicester	St Ivel	620	176
Mozzarella	(US figs)	800	227
Parmesan		760	215
Processed		1,360	385
Roquefort	(US figs)	1,640	465
Stilton (blue)		1,150	326
Stilton (white)	St Ivel	750	212
Wensleydale	St Ivel	450	127
Cheesecake (cooked)	(home-made)	260	74
Cheesecake (frozen)	Sara Lee (approx)	300	85
Cheese sauce: see under Sauce			
Cheese spread		1,170	331
Cherries (cooking)		3	0.8
Cherries (eating)		2	0.5
Cherries, glacé		65	18
Chestnuts (fresh)		11	3.1
Chewing gum	(US figs)	trace	trace

Product	Brand/comments	Na (mg/100g)	Na (mg/oz)
Chicken (meat only)		81	23
Chicken (weighed with bones)		40–50	11–14
Chicken and vegetable pie (frozen)	Findus	659	187
Chicken pie (frozen)	Birds Eye	450	127
Chicken pie (frozen)	Findus	1,926	546
Chicken supreme (frozen)	Birds Eye	390	110
Chick peas (dried)		40	11
Chicory		7	1.9
Chili con carne (canned, with beans)	(US brands)	425–530	120–50
Chili powder (pure)		trace	trace
Chili seasoning	Schwartz	3,660	1,036
Chocolate, drinking (powder)	Cadbury's	294	83
Chocolate, fruit & nut	Cadbury's	110	31
Chocolate, milk	Aero	90	25
Chocolate, milk	Cadbury's	120	34
Chocolate, milk	Galaxy	159	45
Chocolate, plain (sweetened)	Cadbury's Bournville	22	6.2
Chocolate Cream	Fry's	45	13
Chocolate spread	Cadbury's	410	116
Chow mein (dehydrated)	Vesta	420	119
Christmas pudding	(home-made)	240	68
Chutney: see under Pickles			
Cinnamon	(US figs)	8	2.2
Cloves		trace	trace
'Coat and Cook' (various flavours)	Homepride	3,580–5,310	1,014–1,504
Cob nuts: see Hazel nuts			

Product	Brand/comments	Na (mg/100g)	Na (mg/oz)
Cockles (boiled)		3,520	997
Cocoa powder	Cadbury's Bournville	948	269
Coconut (dessicated)		28	7.9
Coconut (fresh)		17	4.8
Coco Pops	Kellogg's	800	227
Cod, dried and salted	(US figs; approx)	8,000	2,270
Cod, dried and salted (soaked and boiled)		400	113
Cod (fresh or frozen)		77	22
Cod (smoked)		1,170	331
Cod in various sauces	Birds Eye	240–400	68–113
Cod liver oil		trace	trace
Cod's roe (fried)		130	37
Cod's roe, smoked	Marina	275	78
Cod steak in breadcrumbs (frozen)	Findus	234	66
Cod steak in crisp crunch crumb (frozen)	Birds Eye	510	144
Cod steaks, battered (frozen)	Findus	612	173
Cod steaks in cheese sauce (frozen)	Findus	258	73
Cod steaks in parsley sauce (frozen)	Findus	168	48
Coffee-Mate	Carnation	146	41
Coleslaw	Eden Vale	347	98
Coleslaw	Mattessons	303	86
Coleslaw	St Ivel	150	42
Coleslaw vinaigrette	Eden Vale	272	77
Coleslaw vinaigrette	Mattessons	318	90
Coleslaw vinaigrette	St Ivel	330	93

Product	Brand/comments	Na (mg/100g)	Na (mg/oz)
Coley (Saithe) (fresh or frozen)		73	20
Complan (natural)	Farley/Glaxo	350	99
Complan (flavoured)	Farley/Glaxo	340–80	96–107
Cooking fat		trace	trace
'Cook-in-Sauce': Chilli	Homepride	880	249
Tomato and onion	Homepride	850	241
other flavours	Homepride	400–730	113–207
Coriander		trace	trace
Corn, sweet (canned)	(average)	310	88
Corn, sweet (canned)	Del Monte	205	58
Corn, sweet (fresh or frozen)		1	0.3
Corned beef (canned)	(average)	950	269
Corned beef (canned)	Fray Bentos	1,400	397
Corn Flakes	Kellogg's	1,180	334
Corn Flakes, Crunchy Nut	Kellogg's	760	215
Cornflour		52	15
Cornish pastie	(average)	590	167
Cornish pastie	Pork Farms	390	110
Cornish pastie (frozen)	Findus	414	117
Corn syrup	(US figs)	68	19
Cottage pie (frozen)	Findus	479	136
Country Store	Kellogg's	390	110
Courgettes (fresh)		trace	trace
Courgettes, sliced (frozen)	Birds Eye	20	5.7
Crab (meat only)		370	105
Crab meat (canned)	(average)	550	156
Crackers: Cheddars	Crawford's	479	136
Cheeselets	Peak Frean	1,391	394

Product	Brand/comments	Na (mg/100g)	Na (mg/oz)
Cheese Ritz	Nabisco	834	236
Cream	(average)	610	172
Cream	Crawford's	490	139
Cream	Jacobs	532	151
Krackawheat	Crawford's	822	233
Ritz	Nabisco	577	163
Tuc	Crawford's	1,067	302
Cranberries		2	0.6
Cream, double (fresh)		27	7.6
Cream, single (fresh)		42	12
Cream, soured (fresh)	St Ivel	40	11
Cream, sterilized (canned)		56	16
Cream, whipped (fresh)		34	9.6
Cream of tartar		trace	trace
Cress	(US figs)	10	2.8
Crispbread: see under brand names			
Crisps: see Potato crisps			
Crumpets	Mother's Pride	820	232
Crunchie	Cadbury's	360	102
Cucumber (fresh)		13	3.7
Cucumber (pickled)	(US figs)	700–2,000	198–566
Cucumber spread	Heinz	720	204
Currants (dried)		20	5.7
Curry and rice with beef (dehydrated)	Batchelors	280	79
Curry and rice with chicken (dehydrated)	Vesta	210	59
Curry Mixes: Korma	Colman's	2,400	680
Madras	Colman's	1,300	368
Tandoori	Colman's	9,500	2,691
Vindaloo	Colman's	3,000	850
Curry powder	(average)	450	127

Product	Brand/comments	Na (mg/100g)	Na (mg/oz)
Custard (as served)	(average)	76	21
Custard (as served; canned)	Ambrosia	52	15
Custard powder (dry weight)		320	91
Custard tart	(home-made)	250	71

Product	Brand/comments	Na (mg/100g)	Na (mg/oz)
Damsons (fresh)		2	0.6
Dandelion leaves (raw)		76	22
Dates (pitted, dried)		5	1.4
Dogfish: see Rock salmon			
Dolly Mixture	Bassetts	18	5.1
Doughnut	(average)	60	17
Doughnut (jam)	Mother's Pride	290	82
Dripping, beef (fat only)		5	1.4
Duck (meat only)		110	31
Duck (meat, fat and skin)		77	22
Dumpling	(home-made)	400	113
Dumpling mix	Lyons-Tetley	650	184
Dutch Crispbake	Nabisco	276	78

Product	Brand/comments	Na (mg/100g)	Na (mg/oz)
Eclairs, chocolate		160	45
Eel (fresh)		89	25
Egg (dried whole)		520	147
Egg (whole)		140	40
Egg custard	(home-made)	78	22
Egg white		190	54
Egg yolk		50	14
Endive		10	2.8
Energen Crispbread		610	173
Energen Rolls		650	184

Product	Brand/comments	Na (mg/100g)	Na (mg/oz)
Faggots	(average)	820	232
Farex	Farley	10	2.8
Farex Fingers	Farley	70	20
Farlene	Farley	35	9.9
Figs, dried (raw)		87	25
Figs, fresh or canned		2	0.6
Fish : Double Decker (frozen)	Findus	1,238	351
Fish cakes (frozen)	(average)	480	136
Fish cakes (frozen)	Findus	431	122
Fish fingers (frozen)	(average)	320	91
Fish fingers (cod, frozen)	Birds Eye	510	144
Fish fingers (cod, frozen)	Findus	368	104
Fish fingers (haddock, frozen)	Findus	360	102
— see also entries for individual types of fish			
Fish paste	(average)	600	170
Flan, egg, cheese and bacon (frozen)	Findus	468	132
Flounder	(US figs)	70	20
Flour, plain (white or brown)		2–4	0.6–1.1
Flour, rye		1	0.3
Flour, self-raising	(approx)	350	99
Flour mix, low-protein	Rite-Diet	10	2.8
Frankfurters: see under Sausages			
French dressing	(home-made)	960	272
French dressing	Heinz	760	215

Product	Brand/comments	Na (mg/100g)	Na (mg/oz)
Frosties	Kellogg's	670	190
Fruit gums	Rowntrees	45	13
Fruit pastilles	Rowntrees	70	20
Fruit pie (individual)	(average)	210	59
Fruit pie (pastry top)	(home-made)	110	31
Fruit pie filling (canned)	(average)	30	8
Fruit salad (canned)	(average)	2	0.6
Fudge (chocolate-coated)	Cadbury's	200	57

Product	Brand/comments	Na (mg/100g)	Na (mg/oz)
Gammon: see under Bacon, Ham			
Garlic	(US figs; approx)	10	2.8
Garlic Salt	Schwartz	29,115	8,248
Gelatine	(US figs)	27	7.6
Gherkins (pickled)	Haywards	750	212
Ginger (ground)		34	9.6
Glucose (liquid)		150	42
Golden Oaties	Quaker	530	150
Golden Syrup	(average)	270	76
Goose (roasted)		150	42
Gooseberries		2	0.6
Grapefruit (canned)		10	2.8
Grapefruit (fresh)		1	0.3
Grape-Nuts		660	187
Grapes		2	0.6
Gravy Pot gravy concentrate	Colmans	4,500	1,275
Greengages		1	0.3
Grouse (meat only; roasted)		96	18
Grouse (weighed with bones; roasted)		63	18
Greens, spring: see Spring greens			
Guavas (canned)		7	2

Product	Brand/comments	Na (mg/100g)	Na (mg/oz)
Haddock, smoked (steamed)	(average)	1,220	346
Haddock fillets (fresh or frozen)		120	34
Haggis (boiled)	(average)	770	218
Hake	(US figs)	74	21
Halibut		84	24
Ham (boiled)	Pork Farms	800	227
Ham (canned)	(average)	1,250	354
Ham (roasted)	Pork Farms	1,000	282
Ham, honey roast	Mattessons	984	279
Ham and pork, chopped (canned)	(average)	1,090	309
Hamburger: see Beefburger			
Hare (stewed)		40	11
Harvest Crunch	Quaker	17	4.8
Harvest Crunch, bran and apple	Quaker	15	4.2
Harvest Crunch Bar, almond and honey	Quaker	111	31
Harvest Crunch Bar, peanut	Quaker	17	4.8
Hazel nuts		1	0.3
Heart, lamb's		140	40
Heart, ox		95	27
Heart, pig		80	23
Heart, sheep's (roasted)		150	42
Hermesetas: see under Saccharine			
Herring (fresh)		67	19
Herring, smoked: see Bloaters, Kippers			
Herring, pickled (rollmop)	Marina	1,700	481
Herring roe (fried)		87	25

Product	Brand/comments	Na (mg/100g)	Na (mg/oz)
Honey		7–10	2.0–2.8
Horlicks tablets	Beechams	330	93
Horse meat		175	49
Horseradish		8	2.3
Horseradish sauce	Colman's	400	113
Hula Hoops	KP	1,550–710	439–84

Product	Brand/comments	Na (mg/100g)	Na (mg/oz)
Ice cream (dairy)		80	23
Ice cream (non-dairy)		70	20

Product	Brand/comments	Na (mg/100g)	Na (mg/oz)
Jaffa Cakes	McVitie's	12	3.4
Jams: Apricot	Chivers	8	2.3
Apricot	Hartley's	95	27
Blackcurrant	Chivers	60	17
Blackcurrant	Hartley's	160	45
Plum	Hartley's	120	34
Raspberry	Chivers	32	9.1
Raspberry	Hartley's	130	37
Strawberry	Chivers	8	2.3
Strawberry	Hartley's	75	21
Jam tarts	(home-made)	230	65
Jam tarts	Mr Kipling	164	46
Jelly babies	Bassetts	26	7.4
Jelly, dessert, as served: (made with water)	(average)	6	1.7
(made with milk)	(average)	27	7.6
Jelly, dessert, as sold		65–250	18–71

Product	Brand/comments	Na (mg/100g)	Na (mg/oz)
Kale	(US figs)	110	31
Ketchup, tomato	(average)	1,120	317
Ketchup, tomato	Daddies	1,336	378
Ketchup, tomato	Heinz	1,450	411
Kidney, lamb's		220	62
Kidney, ox		180	51
Kidney, pig's		190	54
Kippers, baked	(average)	990	280
Kippers, fillets (frozen)	Findus	727	206
Kit Kat	Rowntrees	105	30
Kohlrabi leaves	(US figs)	10	2.8
Kohlrabi root	(US figs)	37	10

Product	Brand/comments	Na (mg/100g)	Na (mg/oz)
Lamb, fat		36	10
Lamb, lean		88	25
Lard		2	0.6
Lasagne (frozen)	Findus	369	104
Laverbread		560	159
Leeks		9	2.5
Lemon (whole)		6	1.7
Lemon cheese	Hartley's	162	46
Lemon curd	(average)	65	18
Lemon curd	(home-made)	150	42
Lemon curd	Gales	80	23
Lemon curd	Hartley's	181	51
Lemon meringue pie	(home-made)	200	57
Lentils (dried)		36	10
Lettuce		9	2.5
Lime (whole)		2	0.6
Ling	(steamed)	120	34
Lion Bar	Rowntrees	180	51
Liquorice allsorts		75	21
Liver, calves'		93	26
Liver, chicken		85	24
Liver, lamb's		76	21
Liver, ox		81	23
Liver, pig's		87	25
Liver sausage	(average)	860	244
Lobster (meat only)		330	93
Loganberries (canned)		1	0.3
Loganberries (fresh)		3	0.8
Low-fat spread	(typical)	690	195
Low-fat spread	Outline	500	142
Lumpfish roe (caviar-style)	Marina	2,750	779
Luncheon meat	(average)	1,050	297

Product	Brand/comments	Na (mg/100g)	Na (mg/oz)
Lychees (canned)		2	0.6
Lychees (fresh)		3	0.8

Product	Brand/comments	Na (mg/100g)	Na (mg/oz)
Macaroni (raw)		26	7.4
Macaroni (raw) (low-protein)	Rite-Diet	15	4.2
Macaroni cheese	Heinz	605	171
Macaroni pudding, creamed	Ambrosia	60	17
Macaroons	Mr Kipling	53	15
Mace (ground)		45	13
Mackerel (fresh)	(average)	130	37
Mackerel (smoked)	no exact figs but very high		
Mackerel fillets in oil or tomato sauce (canned)	Marina	590	167
MacVita	McVitie's	720	204
Maltesers		252	71
Mandarin oranges (canned)		9	2.5
Mango (canned)		3	0.8
Mango (fresh)		7	2
Maple syrup		10–15	2.9–4.2
Margarine	(average)	800	227
Margarine, in general	Van den Berghs brands	920–1,000	261–83
Margarine, Blue Band	Van den Berghs	690	195
Margarine, Flora	Van den Berghs	700	198
Margarine, Krona Export	Van den Berghs	500	142
Margarine, Tomor	Van den Berghs	690	195
— see also Low-fat spread			
Marmalade, lemon (shred)	Chivers	143	40
Marmalade, lemon and lime	Roses	120	34
Marmalade, lime	Roses	170	48

Product	Brand/comments	Na (mg/100g)	Na (mg/oz)
Marmalade, orange	Hartley's	42	12
Marmalade, orange	Roses	150	42
Marmalade, orange (shred)	Chivers	125	35
Marmalade, orange (thick cut)	Chivers	155	44
Marmite		4,500	1,275
Marrow (vegetable)		1	0.3
Mars bar		206	58
Marzipan	(home-made)	13	3.7
Matchmakers	Rowntrees (approx)	55	15
Matzo meal	Rakusen	17	4.9
Matzos: see under Biscuits			
Mayonnaise	(home-made)	360	102
Mayonnaise (low-caloric)	Heinz Slimway	745	211
Meat paste	(average)	740	210
Meat tenderizer	Schwartz	39,055	11,064
Medlars		6	1.7
Melon, cantaloupe		14	4
Melon, honeydew		20	5.7
Melon, water-		4	1.1
Meringues (without cream)	(average)	110	31
Meringues (frozen)	Sara Lee	30	8.5
Milk, condensed, sweetened (skimmed)		180	51
Milk, condensed, sweetened (whole)		130	37
Milk, dried (skimmed)	(average)	550	156
Milk, dried (whole)		440	125
Milk, dried	Five Pints	320	91

Product	Brand/comments	Na (mg/100g)	Na (mg/oz)
Milk, dried	Marvel	573	162
Milk, evaporated, unsweetened	(average)	180	51
Milk, evaporated, unsweetened	Carnation	161	46
Milk, fresh (skimmed)	(average)	52	15
Milk, fresh (whole)		35–90	9.9–25
Milk, goat's		40	11
Milk, human (10 days after childbirth)		25	7.1
Milk, human (1 month after childbirth)		14	4
Milk, sheep's		33	9.3
Milky Way		133	38
Mincemeat	(average)	140	40
Mincemeat	Hartley's	353	100
Mince pies	Mr Kipling	151	43
Mint jelly	Colman's	400	113
Mints, After Eight	Rowntrees	20	5.7
Mints, Glacier	Fox's	35	9.9
— see also Peppermints			
Mint sauce (as sold)	Colman's	2,000	567
Mint sauce	Pan Yan	975	276
Molasses		15–90	4.2–26
Monosodium glutamate		13,610	3,855
Mousse (frozen; various flavours)	Findus	32–82	9.1–23
MSG: see Monosodium glutamate			
Muesli	(average)	180	51
— see also under brand names			
Muffins	Mother's Pride	220	62
Mulberries		2	0.6

Product	Brand/comments	Na (mg/100g)	Na (mg/oz)
Mullet		94	27
Mushrooms (fresh)		9	2.5
Mushrooms (canned)	(US figs)	400–75	113–34
Mussels		290	82
Mussels, in brine (canned)	Marina	472	134
Mustard (prepared): American	(average)	1,300	368
Mustard (prepared): Dijon	Colman's	3,900	1,105
Mustard (prepared): English	Colman's	3,400	963
Mustard (prepared): German	Colman's	2,400	680
Mustard (prepared): Meaux	Colman's	3,300	935
Mustard (prepared): Mild English	Colman's	2,000	566
Mustard and cress		19	5.4
Mustard powder	Colman's	40	11
Mutton		92	26

Product	Brand/comments	Na (mg/100g)	Na (mg/oz)
Nectarines		9	2.5
Noodles: see Macaroni, Spaghetti			
Nougat	Bassets (approx)	65	18
Nutmeg		14	4
Nuts, mixed (roasted and salted)	KP	380–580	108–64
Nuts, mixed (roasted and salted)	Sun-Pat	420	119

Product	Brand/comments	Na (mg/100g)	Na (mg/oz)
Oatcakes		1,230	348
Oat Krunchies	Quaker	615	174
Oatmeal (raw)		33	9.3
Oil, salad or cooking		trace	trace
Okra (fresh)		7	2
Olives in brine (flesh only)		2,250	637
Olives in brine (weighed with stones)		1,800	510
Onion (fresh)		10	2.8
Onions (pickled; standard)	Haywards	700	198
Onions (pickled; silverskin)	Haywards	450	127
Onions (pickled; silverskin)	Heinz	875	248
Onions, spring		13	3.7
Onion salt	Schwartz	29,100	8,244
Opal Fruits		78	22
Orange		3	0.8
Outline: see under Low-Fat Spread			
Oxo beef drink (concentrate)		5,600	1,586
Oxo cubes, beef		10,500	2,974
Oxo cubes, chicken		12,000	3,399
Oxtail		110	31
Oysters (flesh only)		510	144

Product	Brand/comments	Na (mg/100g)	Na (mg/oz)
Paella, chicken and seafood (frozen)	Birds Eye	650	184
Pancreas: see Sweetbreads			
Pancake	(home-made)	50	14
Pancakes, Scotch	(home-made)	400	113
Pancakes, Scotch	Mother's Pride	270	76
Papaya (pawpaw) (canned)		8	2.2
Paprika		83	23
Parsley		33	9.3
Parsnip		17	4.8
Partridge (roasted; meat only)		100	28
Passion fruit		28	7.9
Pastry, choux (raw)	(home-made)	260	74
Pastry, flaky (raw)	(home-made)	350	99
Pastry, puff (frozen)	Jus-Rol	400–550	113–56
Pastry, shortcrust (raw)	(home-made)	410	116
Pastry, shortcrust (frozen)	Jus-Rol	235–390	66
Pastry, shortcrust mix	Lyons	570	161
Pâté, various flavours	Mattessons	560–830	159–235
Pawpaw: see Papaya			
Peaches (canned in syrup)	(average)	1	0.3
Peaches (canned in syrup)	Del Monte	3	0.8
Peaches (dried)		6	1.7
Peaches (fresh)		3	0.8
Peanut butter	(average)	350	99
Peanut butter	Gales	400	113
Peanut butter	Sun-Pat	365	103
Peanuts (dry roasted)	KP	620	176
Peanuts (raw)		6	1.7
Peanuts (roasted and salted)	(average)	440	125

Product	Brand/comments	Na (mg/100g)	Na (mg/oz)
Peanuts (roasted and salted)	KP	380–580	108–64
Peanuts (roasted and salted)	Sun-Pat (approx)	350	99
Peanuts and raisins	KP	29	8.2
Pears (canned)	(average)	1	0.3
Pears (canned)	Del Monte	5	1.4
Pears (fresh)		3	0.8
Peas (dried)		38	11
Peas (fresh)		.1	0.3
Peas (frozen)		3	0.8
Peas, garden (canned)	(average)	230	65
Peas, garden (canned)	Hartley's	259	73
Peas, garden (canned)	Del Monte	288	81
Peas, mushy (canned)	Batchelors	330	93
Peas, processed (canned)	(average)	330	93
Peas, processed (canned)	Batchelors	430	122
Peas, processed (canned)	Hartley's	309	87
Peas, red pigeon		29	8.2
Pepper, black or white		7	2
Pepper, chilli	(US figs)	18	5.0
Pepper, green		2	0.6
Peppermints	Polo	10	2.8
Peppermints	Trebor	10	2.8
Pheasant (meat only; roasted)		100	28
Piccalilli	(average)	1,200	340
Piccalilli	Haywards	1,700	481
Piccalilli	Heinz	1,095	310
Piccalilli	Pan Yan	1,100	312
Piccalilli, sweet	Haywards	1,200	340
Pickles: chutney	(home-made)	130–80	37–51

Product	Brand/comments	Na (mg/100g)	Na (mg/oz)
Farmhouse	Pan Yan	1,300	368
Military	Haywards	1,500	425
Original	Pan Yan	2,500	708
Ploughman's	Heinz	1,390	394
sweet	(average)	1,700	481
— see also individual vegetables (eg, Onions)			
Picnic bar	Cadbury's	140	40
Pigeon (meat only; roasted)		110	31
Pilchards in tomato sauce (canned)	S. African (av)	370	105
Pineapple (canned)		1	0.3
Pineapple (fresh)		2	0.6
Pistachio nuts (salted)	(US figs)	112	32
Pizza, crispy-base (various flavours; frozen)	Findus	512–58	145–58
Pizza, French-bread (various flavours; frozen)	Findus	540–84	153–65
Plaice, filleted		120	34
Plantain (green)		1	0.3
Plums (fresh)		2	0.6
Polony	(average)	870	246
Pomegranate	(approx)	2.5	0.7
Pontefract cakes	Bassetts	128	36
Popcorn (salted)	(US figs – approx)	1,600	453
Popcorn (sweet, unsalted)	(US figs)	3	0.8
Pork (fresh; fat)		38	10
Pork (fresh; lean)		76	21
Pork (salt)	(US figs)	1,200– 2,900	340–821
Pork pie	(average)	720	204
Pork roll, stuffed	Tyne Brand	780	221

Product	Brand/comments	Na (mg/100g)	Na (mg/oz)
Porridge (served as instructed)		580	164
Porridge, instant: see Ready Brek, Warm Start			
Porridge oats: see Oatmeal			
Potassium chloride (salt substitute)		trace	trace
Potassium glutamate (MSG substitute)		trace	trace
Potato, instant (powder)	(average)	1,190	337
Potato, instant (powder)	Cadbury's Smash	1,180	334
Potato, instant (powder)	Yeoman	1,100	312
Potato, instant (made as directed)	(average)	260	74
Potato, instant (made as directed)	Cadbury's Smash	228	64
Potato, instant (made as directed)	Yeoman – made with water	195	55
Potato, instant (made as directed)	Yeoman – made with milk	230	65
Potato, instant, with onions (powder)	Yeoman	1,700	481
Potato, instant, with onions (made as directed)	Yeoman	330	93
Potato chips (frozen)	(average)	25	7.1
Potato chips (frozen)	Birds Eye	40	11
Potato chips, oven-ready (frozen)	Findus	25	7.1
Potato chips, oven-ready (frozen)	McCain	74	21
Potato crisps (mixed)	(average)	550	156
Potato crisps (ready salted)	KP	480–680	136–93
Potatoes, croquette (frozen)	Findus	270	76

Product	Brand/comments	Na (mg/100g)	Na (mg/oz)
Potatoes, new (canned)	(average)	260	74
Potatoes, new (canned)	Hartley's	269	76
Potatoes, new (canned)	Del Monte	357	101
Potatoes, new (canned)	Yeoman	330	93
Potatoes, new (fresh; boiled)	(average)	41	12
Potatoes, old	(average)	71	20
Potato salad (ready-made)	Eden Vale	433	123
Potato salad (ready-made)	Heinz	480	136
Potato salad (ready-made)	Mattessons (approx)	252	71
Potato sticks	KP	480–680	136–93
Potato waffles	Birds Eye	310	88
Prawn cocktail/salad (ready-made)	Eden Vale	385	109
Prawn cocktail/salad (ready-made)	Mattessons (approx)	550	156
Prawns (fresh; boiled)		1,590	450
Pretzels	(US figs)	1,100–3,160	312–895
Prunes (canned)	Del Monte	trace	trace
Prunes (dried)		12	3.4
Puffa Puffa Rice	Kellogg's	160	45
Puffed Wheat	Quaker	4	1.1
Pumpernickel: see under Bread			
Pumpkin		1	0.3

Product	Brand/comments	Na (mg/100g)	Na (mg/oz)
Quail	(US figs; approx)	40	11
Queen of puddings	(home-made)	150	42
Quick lunch (various flavours)	KP	3,200–8,100	906–2,295
Quinces		3	0.8

Product	Brand/comments	Na (mg/100g)	Na (mg/oz)
Rabbit (meat only)		67	19
Radishes		59	17
Raisins (dried)		52	15
Raspberries (canned)		4	1.1
Raspberries (fresh or frozen)		3	0.8
Ravioli in tomato sauce (canned)	Heinz	715	202
Ready Brek	Lyons	40	11
Redcurrants		2	0.6
Refreshers	Trebor	1,000	283
Relishes: Barbeque	Bicks	619	175
Corn	Bicks	446	126
Cucumber (Cubits)	Bicks	370	105
Hamburger	Bicks	479	136
Hot Dog Mild Mustard	Bicks	802	227
Mild Chili	Bicks	446	126
Onion	Bicks	411	116
Revels		163	46
Rhubarb (fresh)		2	0.6
Rice (raw)		6	1.7
Rice, beef flavour	Batchelors	460	130
Rice, chicken flavour	Batchelors	500	142
Rice, mixed vegetable	Batchelors	450	127
Rice Krispies	Kellogg's	1,130	320
Rice pudding (canned)	(average)	50	14
Rice pudding (canned)	Ambrosia	110	31
Rice pudding, creamed (canned)	Ambrosia	51	14
Ricicles	Kellogg's	940	266

Product	Brand/comments	Na (mg/100g)	Na (mg/oz)
Rock salmon (dogfish) (fried in batter)		290	82
Rolo	Rowntrees	250	71
Rusks	Oster	110	31
Rusks, low-sodium	Farley's	5.3	1.5
Ryking, brown rye		432	122
Ryking, golden wheat		628	178
Ryking, other types		471	133
Ryvita (original)		220	62
Ryvita, brown		440	125
Ryvita, salt-free		3	0.8

Product	Brand/comments	Na (mg/100g)	Na (mg/oz)
Saccharine (pure)		nil	nil
Saccharine (soluble)	Hermesetas	9,913	2,808
Saccharine (soluble) per tablet	Hermesetas	1.6mg	
Sage		19	5.4
Sago (raw)		3	0.8
Saithe: see Coley			
Salad cream	(average)	840	238
Salad cream	Heinz	1,200	340
— see also French Dressing, Mayonnaise			
Salami	(average)	1,850	524
Salmon (canned, red)	(average)	570	161
Salmon (fresh)		98	28
Salmon (smoked)		1,880	532
Salsify (boiled)		8	2.3
Salt		38,850	11,006
Salt substitute (low sodium)	(typical)	19,415	5,500
Salt substitute (sodium-free)		trace	trace
Sandwich Spread	Heinz	1,000	283
Sardines in oil (canned)	(fish only)	650	184
Sardines in oil (canned)	(fish and oil)	540	153
Sardines in tomato sauce (canned)	(average)	700	198
Sauce, apple	Colman's dry mix	1,800	510
Sauce, apple	Heinz canned	5	1.5
Sauce, apple	Pan Yan	40	11
Sauce, barbecue	Colman's dry mix	5,100	1,445
Sauce, bread	(home-made)	490	139
Sauce, bread	Colman's dry mix	3,000	850
Sauce, brown	Daddies	1,454	412
Sauce, brown	HP	1,440	408

Product	Brand/comments	Na (mg/100g)	Na (mg/oz)
Sauce, brown	HP Fruity	1,415	401
Sauce, brown	OK Fruity	1,200	340
Sauce, brown	OK Spicy	1,400	397
Sauce, cheese	(home-made)	450	127
Sauce, cheese	Colman's dry mix	3,900	1,105
Sauce, cranberry	Ocean Spray	2	0.6
Sauce, cranberry (jellied)	Ocean Spray	28	7.9
Sauce, cranberry and orange	Ocean Spray	6	1.7
Sauce, mint: see Mint sauce			
Sauce, onion	(home-made)	440	125
Sauce, onion	Colman's dry mix	3,200	906
Sauce, parsley	Colman's dry mix	3,700	1,048
Sauce, soy: see Soy sauce			
Sauce, sweet and sour	Colman's dry mix	5,200	1,473
Sauce, tartare	Colman's	800	227
Sauce, tomato: see Ketchup			
Sauce, white (savoury)	(home-made)	410	116
Sauce, white (savoury)	Colman's dry mix	2,600	736
Sauce, white (sweet)	(home-made)	110	31
Sauce, Worcestershire	Lea & Perrins (approx)	1,300	368
Sauerkraut		740	210
Sausage, garlic	Mattessons (approx)	630	178
Sausage roll	(home-made)	550–80	156–64
Sausage roll	Pork farms	660	187
Sausage roll (frozen)	Findus	503	142
Sausages, beef	(average)	810	229
Sausages, frankfurter (canned/packets)	(average)	980	278
Sausages, frankfurter	Mattessons	550	156

Product	Brand/comments	Na (mg/100g)	Na (mg/oz)
Sausages, pork	(average)	760	215
Sausages, pork	Pork Farms	570	161
Sausages, pork and beef	Pork Farms	630	178
Sausages, turkey	Bernard Matthews	900	255
— see also individual types not listed above			
Saveloy	(average)	890	252
Scallops (steamed)	weighed (without shell)	270	76
Scampi (frozen, fried)	(average)	380	108
Scones	(home-made)	800	227
Scones	Mother's Pride	540	153
Scotch pancakes: see under Pancakes			
Seakale (boiled)		4	1.1
Seasoning, barbecue	Schwartz	10,990	3,113
Seasoning, chicken	Schwartz	29,875	8,463
Seasoning, chili	Schwartz	3,660	1,037
Seasoning, grill	Schwartz	16,500	4,674
Seasoning, pork	Schwartz	17,890	5,068
Seasoning, salad	Schwartz	11,480	3,252
Seasoning, sandwich	Schwartz	20,340	5,762
Seasoning, steak	Schwartz	15,790	4,473
Seasoning salt	Schwartz	20,245	5,735
Semolina (raw)		12	3.4
Semolina pudding, creamed	Ambrosia	62	17
Sesame seeds		60	17
Shad		54	15
Shallots		11	3.1
Shepherd's pie (frozen)	Findus	463	131
Sherbert Lemons	Trebor	300	85
Sherbert powder	Bassetts	1,257	356

Product	Brand/comments	Na (mg/100g)	Na (mg/oz)
Shortbread	(home-made)	270	76
Shortbread	Crawford's	302	85
Shortening: see Cooking Fat			
Shredded Wheat	Nabisco	12	3.4
Shreddies	Nabisco	569	161
Shrimps (canned)		980	277
Shrimps (fresh, boiled)		3,840	1,088
Sild in oil (canned)	(US figs)	170	48
Skate (fried in batter)		140	40
Slender (various flavours)	Carnation; dry weight	353	100
Smarties	Rowntrees	45	13
Smelts (fried)		148	42
Snapper, red	(US figs)	67	19
Sodium ascorbate (form of vitamin C)		11,616	4,100
Sodium benzoate (preservative)		15,972	5,638
Sodium bicarbonate (baking soda)		27,400	7,760
Sodium carbonate monohydrate		37,097	10,509
Sodium chloride (common salt)		38,850	11,005
Sodium nitrite (preservative – for curing meat)		33,333	9,443
Sodium phosphate (powder form)		17,165	4,862
Sodium propionate		23,958	6,787
Sodium sulphite (preservative)		36,508	10,342
Sole, lemon		95	27
Sorbet, lemon	Wall's	21	5.9

Product	Brand/comments	Na (mg/100g)	Na (mg/oz)
Soups: Beef and tomato (dried – made as directed)	Batchelors Cup-a-Soup	430	122
Beef broth (canned)	Heinz	510	144
Chicken, thick (dried – made as directed)	Batchelors 5-Min	380	108
Chicken noodle (dried – made as directed)	(average)	370	105
Chicken noodle (dried – made as directed)	Batchelors 5-Min	390	110
Cream of celery (canned)	Heinz	520	147
Cream of chicken (canned)	(average)	460	130
Cream of chicken (canned)	Heinz	520	147
Cream of chicken (canned; condensed – made as directed)	(average)	350	99
Cream of mushroom (canned)	(average)	470	133
Cream of mushroom (canned)	Heinz	490	139
Cream of tomato (canned)	(average)	460	130
Cream of tomato (canned)	Heinz	720	203
Cream of tomato (canned; condensed – made as directed)	(average)	410	116

Product	Brand/comments	Na (mg/100g)	Na (mg/oz)
Golden vegetable (dried – made as directed)	Batchelors Cup-a-Soup	400	113
Lentil	(home-made)	190	54
Lentil (canned)	Heinz	520	147
Minestrone (canned)	Heinz	685	194
Minestrone (canned)	Heinz Big Soup	550	156
Minestrone (dried – made as directed)	(average)	430	122
Minestrone (dried – made as directed)	Batchelors 5-Min	270	76
Mulligatawny (canned)	Heinz	465	132
Oxtail (canned)	(average)	440	125
Oxtail (canned)	Heinz	520	147
Oxtail (dried – made as directed)	(average)	400	113
Oxtail (dried – made as directed)	Batchelors Cup-a-Soup	590	167
Pea, thick (dried – made as directed)	Batchelors 5-Min	330	93
Pea and ham (canned)	Heinz	480	136
Scotch broth (canned)	Heinz	670	190
Tomato (dried – made as directed)	(average)	390	110
Tomato (dried – made as directed)	Batchelors 5-Min	350	99
Vegetable (canned)	(average)	500	142
Vegetable (canned)	Heinz	520	147
Vegetable (canned)	Heinz Big Soup	459	130

Product	Brand/comments	Na (mg/100g)	Na (mg/oz)
Vegetable (canned)	Heinz Low-Calorie	630	178
Vegetable, spring (canned)	Heinz	440	125
Soya bean curd (tofu)	(US figs)	6.7	1.9
Soya beans (dried)	(US figs)	4	1.1
Soya beans (canned)	(US figs)	237	67
Soya flour		1	0.3
Soy sauce	(US figs)	7,340	2,080
Spaghetti (raw)		5	1.4
Spaghetti (boiled)		2	0.6
Spaghetti bolognaise (canned)	Heinz	410	116
Spaghetti in tomato sauce (canned)	(average)	500	142
Spaghetti in tomato sauce (canned)	Heinz	490	139
Spangles		72	20
Special K	Kellogg's	980	278
Spinach (canned)	Del Monte	338	96
Spinach (fresh; boiled)		120	34
Spinach (frozen)	Findus	53–7	15–16
Sponge pudding (steamed)	(home-made)	310	88
Sponge pudding, chocolate (canned)	Heinz	250	71
Sponge pudding, treacle (canned)	Heinz	350	99
Sprats, fresh (fried)		130	37
Sprats, smoked (grilled)		847	240
Spring greens (boiled)		10	2.8
Steak: see Beef			
Steak, stewed with gravy (canned)	(average)	380	108

Product	Brand/comments	Na (mg/100g)	Na (mg/oz)
Steak and kidney pie	(home-made)	680	193
Steak and kidney pie (canned)	Pork Farms	500	142
Steak and kidney pie (canned)	Tyne Brand	540	153
Steak and kidney pie (frozen)	Birds Eye	430	122
Steak and kidney pie (frozen)	Findus	422	119
Steak and kidney pie filling (canned)	Tyne Brand	580	164
Steak and kidney pudding (canned)	Tyne Brand	450	127
Steak and onion pie filling (canned)	Tyne Brand	400	113
Steak pie filling, stewed (canned)	Tyne Brand	410	116
Stock cubes, beef	Fray Bentos	19,913	5,641
Stock cubes, chicken	Fray Bentos	20,300	5,750
Stock cubes, vegetable and chicken	Bovril	13,300	3,768
Stock cubes, vegetable and meat	Bovril	12,400	3,512
Strawberries (fresh or frozen)		2	0.6
Strawberries (canned)		7	2.0
Sturgeon (steamed)	(US figs)	108	30
Suet (block)		21	5.9
Suet (shredded)		trace	trace
Suet pudding (steamed)	(home-made)	470	133
Sugar, brown	(US figs)	24–30	6.8–8.5
Sugar, Demerara		6	1.7
Sugar, white		trace	trace
Sugar Puffs	Quaker	9	2.5

Product	Brand/comments	Na (mg/100g)	Na (mg/oz)
Sugar Smacks	Kellogg's	10	2.8
Sultana Bran	Kellogg's	710	201
Sultanas		53	15
Super Noodles (made as directed)			
Barbecue	Kellogg's	600	170
Chicken	Kellogg's	560	159
Mild Curry	Kellogg's	920	261
Spicy Beef	Kellogg's	1,070	303
Tomato	Kellogg's	740	210
Swedes		52	15
Sweetbreads (pancreas), lamb's		75	21
Sweet corn: see under Corn			
Sweet potatoes (canned)	(US figs)	48	13
Sweet potatoes (fresh)		19	5.4
Sweets, boiled	(average)	25	7.1
Sweets, boiled	Bassetts	43	12
Sweets, boiled	Trebor	150	42

Syrup: see Golden Syrup, Maple Syrup

Product	Brand/comments	Na (mg/100g)	Na (mg/oz)
Tabasco sauce	McIlhenny (US figs)	600	170
Tangerine		2	0.6
Tapioca		4	1.1
Tarragon		trace	trace
Tea-Mate	Carnation	180	51
Tehina	(approx)	400	113
Thyme		trace	trace
Toast, savoury – ham and cheese (frozen)	Findus	630	178
Toast Toppers – various flavours	Heinz	400–720	113–204
Tobacco, chewing	(US figs)	1,610	456
Toffees, mixed	(average)	320	91
Toffees, mixed	Trebor	400	113
Toffees, Toffo	Rowntrees	250	71
Tomatoes (canned)	(average)	29	8.2
Tomatoes (fresh)		3	0.8
Tomato paste or purée (1% salt)		420	119
Tomato paste or purée (unsalted)		20	5.7
Tomato sauce – see Ketchup			
Tongue, lamb and ox (canned)	(average)	1,050	297
Tongue, lamb (fresh, cured)		420	119
Tongue, ox (pickled)		1,210	343
Tongue, sheep (stewed)		80	23
Topic		201	57
Top 'n' Fill – various flavours	Homepride	190–220	54–62
Treacle, black		96	27

Product	Brand/comments	Na (mg/100g)	Na (mg/oz)
— see also Golden syrup			
Treacle tart	(home-made)	360	102
Treacle tart	Mr Kipling	106	30
Treets, peanut		73	21
Treets, toffee		220	62
Tripe (dressed)		46	13
Trout, river (steamed)		88	25
Trout, sea (steamed)		210	59
Tuna in oil, skipjack (canned)		420	119
Tunes		72	20
Turbot	(US figs)	57	16
Turkey (fresh; meat only)		54	15
Turkey (fresh; meat and skin)		49	14
Turkey, breaded steaks	Bernard Matthews	500	142
Turkey Roast – meat	Bernard Matthews	550	156
Turkey Roast – fat	Bernard Matthews	370	105
Turnips		58	16
Turnip tops/greens (boiled)		7	2
Twiglets	Peak Frean	1,492	423
Twix		248	70

Product	Brand/comments	Na (mg/100g)	Na (mg/oz)
Vanilla extract	(US figs)	1	0.3
Veal fillet		110	31
Veal, jellied (canned)		1,190	337
Vegetables, mixed (canned)	Hartley's	306	87
Vegetables, mixed (frozen)	Findus	13	3.7
Vegetables, Garden Mix (frozen)	Findus	58	16
Vegetable salad	Eden Vale	548	155
Vegetable salad (canned)	Heinz	440	125
Venison (roasted)		86	24
Vinegar		20	5.7
Vitawheat, rye	Jacobs	787	223
Vitawheat, standard	Jacobs	799	226

Product	Brand/comments	Na (mg/100g)	Na (mg/oz)
Walnuts (fresh)		3	0.8
Walnuts (pickled)	Epicure	1,260	357
Walnuts (pickled)	Haywards	900	255
Walnut Whip, milk chocolate	Rowntrees (approx)	70	20
Warm Start	Quaker	33	9.3
Watercress		60	17
Water ice: see Sorbet			
Watermelon		trace	trace
Weetabix		375	106
Weetaflakes		300	85
Whale meat	(US figs)	78	22
Wheat flakes	Force (old figs)	695	197
Wheat germ		2	0.6
Whelks (flesh only, boiled)		270	76
Whitebait (floured and fried)		230	65
White currants		2	0.6
White pudding	(average)	370	105
White sauce – see under Sauce			
Whiting (fried)		200	57
Whiting (steamed)		130	37
Wine, 'cooking'	(may contain up to)	600	170
Wine gums	Bassetts	60	17
Winkles (flesh only, boiled)		1,140	323

Product	Brand/comments	Na (mg/100g)	Na (mg/oz)
Yams (boiled)		17	4.8
Yeast, baker's (compressed; fresh)		16	4.5
Yeast, baker's (dried)	(approx)	50	14
Yeast, brewer's	(US figs)	180	51
Yeast extract: see Marmite			
Yoghurt, chocolate	Eden Vale	129	36
Yoghurt, flavoured	(average)	64	18
Yoghurt, fruit	(average)	64	18
Yoghurt, fruit	Ski	68–80	19–23
Yoghurt, fruit	St Ivel	75	21
Yoghurt, hazelnut		70	20
Yoghurt, natural	(average)	76	22
Yoghurt, natural	Eden Vale	129	36
Yoghurt, natural	St Ivel	90	25
Yoghurt dressing	Heinz	825	234
Yorkshire Pudding	(home-made)	600	170

Alcohol and soft drinks

Product	Brand/comments	Na (mg/100ml)*	Na (mg/fl oz)*
Apple juice	Schloer	8	2.3
Apricot nectar	(US figs)	7	2
Beers:bitter (canned)		9	2.5
bitter (draught)		12	3.4
bitter (keg)		8	2.3
brown ale (bottled)		16	4.5
lager (bottled)		4	1.1
mild (draught)		11	3.1
pale ale (bottled)		10	2.8
stout (bottled)		23	6.5
strong ale		15	4.2
Bitter lemon (low-calorie)	Hunts	15	4.2
Bitter lemon (low-calorie)	Schweppes	23	6.5
Bitter lemon (regular)	Hunts	8	2.3
Bitter lemon (regular)	Schweppes	20	5.7
Blackcurrant juice: see Ribena			
Bournvita (powder)		187*	53*
Bovril – see main listing			
Brandy		3	0.8
Buttermilk	(US figs)	50–130	14–37
Cherryade	Corona	13	3.7
Chocolate, hot/drinking (powder)	Cadbury's	294*	83*
Chocolate, hot/drinking (powder – add hot water only)	Carnation	350*	99*
Cider, dry	(average)	7	2
Cider, sweet	(average)	7	2
Coca-Cola		8	2.3

*Except for powders, which are given as mg/100g and mg/oz

Product	Brand/comments	Na (mg/100ml)*	Na (mg/fl oz)*
Cocoa (powder)	Cadbury's Bournville	948*	268*
Coconut milk		110	31
Coffee (roasted beans, ground)		74*	21*
Coffee (instant powder)		41*	12*
Coffee, black (from beans)		trace	trace
Coffee and chicory essence (concentrated)		65	18
C-Vit	Beechams	24	6.8
Gin		1	0.3
Ginger ale, American	Hunts	4	1.1
Ginger ale, American (low-calorie)	Schweppes	7	2
Ginger ale, American (regular)	Schweppes	5	1.4
Ginger ale, dry	Hunts	5	1.4
Ginger ale, dry	Schweppes	3	0.8
Ginger beer	Hunts	5	1.4
Ginger beer	Schweppes	17	4.8
Grapefruit juice (canned)	(average)	3	0.8
Grapefruit juice (canned)	Heinz	5	1.4
Grapefruit juice (canned)	Del Monte	trace	trace
Grape juice (bottled or canned)	(US figs)	2	0.6
Horlicks (powder)		330*	93*
Horlicks, instant (powder)		642*	182*
Lemonade	Hunts	9	2.5

*Except for powders, which are given as mg/100g and mg/oz

Product	Brand/comments	Na (mg/100ml)*	Na (mg/fl oz)*
Lemonade (low-calorie)	Schweppes	19	5.4
Lemonade (regular)	Schweppes	3	0.8
Lemon and lime, sparkling	Zing	21	5.9
Lemon barley water (undiluted)	Corona	23	6.5
Lemon barley water (undiluted)	Robinson's	29	8.2
Lemon juice	Jif	40	11
Lemon juice	PLJ	31	8.8
Lemon juice (fresh)		2	0.6
Lemon squash/drink (undiluted)	Corona	22	6.2
Lemon squash/drink (undiluted)	Idris	23	6.5
Lemon squash/drink (undiluted)	Kia-Ora	19	5.4
Lemon squash/drink (undiluted)	Robinson's	45	12
Lemon squash/drink (undiluted)	Schweppes	90	25
Lemon squash/drink (diabetic, undiluted)	Rose's	21	5.9
Lemon squash/drink (double-concentrated)	Suncrush	193	55
Lime cordial (undiluted)	Corona	18	5.1
Lime cordial (undiluted)	Rose's	13	3.7
Lime cordial (undiluted)	Schweppes	8	2.3
Lucozade		30	8.5
Milk: see main listing			
Milk shake mix (various flavours; powder)	Kellogg's Two Shakes	360–460	102–30

* Except for powders, which are given as mg/100g and mg/oz

Product	Brand/comments	Na (mg/100ml)*	Na (mg/fl oz) *
Orange, sparkling	Corona	7	2
Orange, sparkling	Idris	7	2
Orange, sparkling	Tango	7	2
Orange, sparkling (low-calorie)	Schweppes	25	7.1
Orange, sparkling (regular)	Schweppes	7	2.0
Orange barley water (undiluted)	Robinson's	30	8.4
Orange juice (canned or fresh)		2–5	0.6–1.4
Orange squash/drink (undiluted)	Corona	13	3.7
Orange squash/drink (undiluted)	Idris	23	6.5
Orange squash/drink (undiluted)	Kia-Ora	19	5.4
Orange squash/drink (undiluted)	Robinson's	35	9.9
Orange squash/drink (undiluted)	Schweppes	92	26
Orange squash/drink (diabetic; undiluted)	Rose's	23	6.5
Orange squash/drink (double-concentrated)	Suncrush	39	11
Oxo Beef Drink (concentrated)		5,600	1,586
Ovaltine (powder)		110*	31*
Pepsi-Cola		10	2.8
Pepsi-Cola (low-calorie)		14	3.7
Phospherine Tonic Wine		124	35
Pineapple juice (canned)		1–5	0.3–1.4

*Except for powders, which are given as mg/100g and mg/oz

Product	Brand/comments	Na (mg/100ml)*	Na (mg/fl oz)*
Pomegranate juice		1	0.3
Port		4	1.1
Prune juice	(US figs)	2	0.6
Ribena (undiluted)		25	7.1
Ribena, baby (undiluted)		94	27
Rise and Shine (powder):			
Blackcurrant	Kellogg's	98*	28*
Grapefruit	Kellogg's	271*	77*
Lemon	Kellogg's	37*	10*
Orange	Kellogg's	378*	107*
Pineapple	Kellogg's	261*	74*
Rose-hip syrup (undiluted)		280	79
Rum		2	0.6
Seven-Up		9	2.5
Shandy	Top Deck	10	2.8
Shandy (low-calorie)	Schweppes	19	5.4
Shandy (regular)	Schweppes	6	1.7
Sherry, dry		10	2.8
Sherry, medium		6	1.7
Sherry, sweet		13	3.7
Soda water	Hunts	32	9.1
Soda water	Schweppes	25	7.1
Tea (as drunk)		trace	trace
Tea (leaves)		45*	13*
Tomato juice (canned)	(average)	240	68
Tomato juice (canned)	Heinz	240	68
Tomato juice cocktail	Hunts	188	53

*Except for powders, which are given as mg/100g and mg/oz

Product	Brand/comments	Na (mg/100ml)*	Na (mg/fl oz) *
Tomato juice cocktail	Schweppes	275	78
Tonic water	Hunts	5	1.4
Tonic water (low calorie)	Schweppes	14	4
Tonic water (regular)	Schweppes	1	0.3
Vermouth, dry	(average)	17	4.8
Vermouth, sweet	(average)	28	7.9
Vodka		trace	trace

Water, mineral

Which?, the magazine of the Consumers' Association, reported in 1983 that, of 34 brands of bottled water checked, the three with the highest sodium level were *Apollinaris*, *Saint-Yorre* and *Vichy-Célestins*. Five more – *Badoit*, *Ferranelle*, *Hisar*, *Saint Léger* and *San Pellegrino* – rated 'medium', while the other 26 contained less than 2 mg per 100 ml – and insignificant level in practice.

* Except for powders, which are given as mg/100g and mg/oz

Product	Brand/comments	Na (mg/100ml)*	Na (mg/fl oz)*

Water, tap

Can vary from a trace to 40 mg/100 ml (11 mg/fl oz), but water supplies in Britain are usually quite low in sodium (eg, London water averages 2.5 to 4 mg/100 ml). The main problem is likely to arise where water comes from underground (artesian) sources near the coast. For precise local information, ask your water board or company. Artificially softened water may contain high levels of sodium; do not use a water softener to supply drinking or cooking water.

Product	Brand/comments	Na (mg/100ml)*	Na (mg/fl oz)*
Whisky		trace	trace
Wine, red	(average)	10	2.8
Wine, rosé	(average)	4	1.1
Wine, sparkling	(Champagne)	4	1.1
Wine, white, dry	(average)	4	1.1
Wine, white, medium	(Graves)	21	5.9
Wine, white, sweet	(Sauternes)	13	3.7

Low-sodium cooking

Any serious attempt to reduce your sodium consumption will, apart from cutting out the obvious high-sodium foods listed on the preceding pages, inevitably involve a change in cooking habits and adjustments to favourite recipes. These can be quite traumatic to your palate if instituted abruptly, but many converts to low-salt eating are adamant that, once adjusted, their palate 'grows up' and acquires a new sensitivity to the true flavours of foods.

In the meantime, however, the natural urge is to turn to other food flavourings in order to ginger up your dishes. As you will see from the listings, there are plenty of low-sodium herbs, spices and other flavourings available, with which you can experiment. When you embark on your culinary revolution, make sure that you have ample supplies in the cupboard.

Lemon juice and vinegar are useful standbys with many savoury dishes – especially vegetables and egg dishes respectively – together with garlic and onion (either fresh or powdered), chives and dry mustard (but *not* garlic salt, onion salt or prepared mustard). There are peppers of various colours – white, black and red (both the mild paprika type and the very different cayenne, a form of chilli). Keep supplies of all the classic herbs, too: basil, bay, marjoram, mint, parsley, rosemary, sage, tarragon, thyme and so on. With them all, the fresher they are the better.

If you feel more adventurous, try such Indian spices as cardamom, turmeric, cumin, coriander and fenugreek, which, together with ginger, chilli, cinnamon, mace and others, form the basis of curries and other Indian dishes. There are many more that I have no room to mention here, but I would recommend, first, that you obtain a good book of culinary herbs and spices and, second, that you go on a shopping spree to your local delicatessen or oriental grocers. Experiment using small quantities at first and keeping notes of successes and failures.

Another approach that may appeal is to use a low-sodium salt-substitute in place of ordinary salt. There are fewer of these in Britain than in North America, but one or two brands have appeared, mainly in health-food stores. Such substitutes are generally made with potassium chloride (sometimes calcium or ammonium chloride), and there are two main snags in using them. First, they tend to taste bitter, so that many people find that they prefer to use nothing at all. Secondly, in one or two medical conditions such substitutes can be dangerous, so it is wise to check with your doctor before switching.

You should also remember that 'low salt' does not mean 'no salt', and some substitutes on the market contain common salt (that is, sodium chloride) blended with potassium and/or other salts. The taste may well be better, but unless you keep strict control you may still be consuming large amounts of sodium. For example, if the figure is 50 per cent sodium chloride, a teaspoonful is still equivalent to 1,000 milligrams of sodium. So be very cautious, read the label, and make sure that you are not unwittingly consuming a lot of sodium in disguise.

A small adjustment of habit, apart from banning the salt-cellar and avoiding MSG, baking soda and branded seasonings, is to use only unsalted butter or margarine, both in cooking and on the table. But keep things in perspective. Unless you have been prescribed a very strict low-sodium diet, judicious use of salt where it matters most need not ruin all the good done by your abstention the rest of the time. The important thing is to keep count of your intake and do a little calculating.

For example, if you feel that a quarter-teaspoonful of salt would make all the difference to a family dish, remember that this contains about 500 milligrams of sodium. Divided between four people, that is 125 milligrams each – a substantial part of your daily allowance, perhaps, but quite acceptable so long as you really do keep a check on the rest of your sodium consumption and keep your 'cheating' under strict control.

The two foods that most people would agree most demand such cheating are eggs and potatoes. The former are much easier to take without salt in the form of Spanish omelettes (see below) and suchlike, where onions, tomatoes, mushrooms and green or red peppers spice up the flavour, rather than simply boiled or poached. With potatoes, you will find that new potatoes (like new carrots) taste much better without salt than old, and the waxy varieties better than the floury ones.

Spanish omelette

Serves 2. Sodium per serving: approx 80 mg

2 large eggs
2 tablespoons water
1 onion, chopped
½ green or red pepper, chopped
225 g (8 oz) fresh tomatoes*, blanched, peeled and chopped

50 g (2 oz) mushrooms, chopped
50 g (2 oz) fresh or frozen peas *or* frozen sweet corn
Unsalted butter
Pepper

Brown the onion in a little butter. Add green or red pepper, tomatoes, mushrooms and peas or sweet corn. Stew gently until soft. Beat eggs with water and add pepper to taste. Make omelette in the usual way with the remaining butter. Before it sets, stir in vegetable mixture.

If you wish, you can add a chopped clove of garlic and/or a pinch of cayenne pepper or chilli powder (not chilli seasoning) to the vegetable mixture. On the plate, season if desired with a little vinegar.

*Using canned tomatoes increases sodium to approx 110 mg per serving.

Vegetables

No-salt cooking really does allow the flavour of fresh vegetables to come through unmasked, but you should be careful not to over-cook green vegetables or they will simply taste bland and mushy. However, even the freshest, most delicately cooked vegetables can make dull eating if you do not vary the preparation, so experiment with spices and fresh herbs as garnishes or added in the cooking. Here are a few ideas of combinations to try:

Asparagus (boiled)	– serve with lemon juice, pepper and butter (optional)
Beans (green)	– boil with mint
	– boil with dill and rosemary
	– parboil, then sauté with onion and lemon juice or with onion, garlic and tomato
Broccoli	– boil; serve with sauce of lemon juice, melted butter, paprika and mustard
Brussels sprouts	– boil with nutmeg and caraway seed
Cabbage	– boil with fennel and nutmeg
	– stir-fry with onion and pepper, with or without sour cream
	– boil; sprinkle with vinegar or lemon juice
Cabbage, red	– cook with vinegar and sugar
	– stir-fry with onion, apple, vinegar, redcurrant jelly, nutmeg, clove and pepper
Carrots	– parboil; sauté with butter, sugar and cinnamon, or with onion
	– boil; season with lemon juice, pepper and parsley
Cauliflower	– boil; serve with sauce of lemon juice, melted butter and pepper
Courgettes	– boil; serve with lemon juice, butter and pepper
	– make into ratatouille with green or red pepper, onion, tomato, basil, oregano, parsley
Mushrooms	– sauté with lemon, pepper and either basil or paprika
	– cook in sour cream and paprika, thickened with flour
Peas	– boil with mint or dill
	– boil with sugar and lemon juice
	– parboil; sauté with onion and/or garlic and pepper
Potatoes	– serve with butter and parsley

Rice	– boil with lemon rind, parsley and cumin
	– boil with saffron
Tomatoes	– grill with basil and/or oregano and/or pepper
	– grill with chopped garlic and basil

Baking

The basic rule is always to use plain (not self-raising) flour with sodium-free rising agents where needed. Substitute bicarbonate of potash (potassium bicarbonate; obtainable from a chemist's) for baking soda (bicarbonate of soda). Increase the quantity used by one-quarter.

For baking powder, ask a chemist to make up the following mixture:

50 g cornflour
70 g potassium bicarbonate
100 g cream of tartar
13.5 g tartaric acid

Mix thoroughly and keep in an airtight jar. Increase the quantity used by one-half (ie, use 1½ times the amount of ordinary baking powder specified in the recipe).

And, of course, you should use unsalted butter or vegetable shortening rather than salted margarine when making cakes and pastries. Bread without salt takes some getting used to, but if you forget about buying commercial low-sodium canned bread, the delicious flavour of fresh home-baked bread more than compensates. And if it is not quite fresh, a few minutes in a hot oven will make all the difference.

Proprietary
medicines

Some over-the-counter medicines – in particular (but not solely) effervescent indigestion and similar products – contain significant amounts of sodium, and you should avoid these if you are on a low-sodium diet. A selection of popular products – though not an exhaustive listing – is given below.

Just as with prepared foods, read the labels, and if in doubt ask the pharmacist to recommend a low-sodium alternative. (For example, indigestion products based on aluminium or magnesium hydroxide are generally sodium-free and just as effective.)

Product	Sodium content
Alka Seltzer	445 mg per tablet
Andrews Liver Salt	6,200 mg per 100 g
Andrews Liver Salt for Diabetics	11,600 mg per 100 g
Bismag Powder	13,190 mg per 100 g
Bismag Tablets	41 mg per tablet
BiSoDoL Powder	15,860 mg per 100 g
BiSoDoL Tablets	17 mg per tablet
Boots Alkaline Stomach Powder	3,425 per 100 g
Boots Cold Relief	39 mg per sachet
Boots Dyspepsia Tablets	41 mg per tablet
Boots Gripe Mixture	274 mg per 100 ml (14 mg per 5 ml spoonful)
Boots Health Salt	6,400 mg per 100 g
Boots Indigestion Mixture	1,235 mg per 100 g
Boots Indigestion Tablets	16 mg per tablet
Boots Sparkling Health Salt	15,235 mg per 100 g
Cupal Baby Gripe Mixture	680 mg per 100 ml (34 mg per 5 ml spoonful)
Eno Fruit Salt	15,235 mg per 100 g
Fynnon Salt	36,035 mg per 100 g

Product	Sodium content
Lem–Sip	39 mg per sachet
Setlers	4.8 mg per tablet

The Good Health Guide £5.95

A splendidly illustrated encyclopaedia of the ways you and your family can enjoy healthy and satisfying lives, written by a team of Open University experts with the aim of linking your physical and psychological health to daily choices about the way you live.

'Comprehensive, attractive and lavishly illustrated. Fascinating and compelling . . . really excellent' YORKSHIRE POST

Col James L. Anderson and Martin Cohen
The West Point Fitness and Diet Book £1.20

From the US Army's top experts in physical fitness – a complete conditioning programme for every member of the family, enabling each member to enjoy the best of health and top physical condition whether they're involved in competitive sport, relaxing in retirement, or busy at the office or in the home all day. Includes: the walk/run plan – weight control and nutrition – posture: how to look good – sports for everyone at every age – special fitness for women.

Slimming Magazine's Complete Dieting Revolution £1.50

How to get slim and stay slim – without calorie-counting, without boredom, without fuss, without fasting. The low-fat diet is a complete revolution in nutritional thinking, based on the theory that if you look after the fats, the calories will look after themselves. Tried, tested and approved by the medical profession, pioneered in Britain by *Slimming Magazine*, this is the new blueprint for anyone who wants to get slim and stay that way.

Dr Andrew Stanway
Taking the Rough with the Smooth £1.95

The discovery that foods rich in dietary fibre (roughage) can help prevent the serious diseases of the affluent society has been heralded as the medical breakthrough of the decade. This is the definitive book on the subject written for the general reader.

Mouthwatering high-fibre recipes are included to enable readers to adapt their diets for a happier and healthier life.

Richard Mackarness
Chemical Victims £1.50

A startling new look at how chemicals in the environment are affecting your health. This book, by the bestselling author of *Not All in the Mind*, considers the long-term effects of the synthetic chemicals in our food and water, even in the air we breathe, and whether more and more illness is being caused by man-made pollutants. There are no comfortable answers. Dr Mackarness — widely experienced in clinical research into food and chemical allergies — suggests that 'problem' patients are not being helped by more and more surgery and drugs; careful avoidance of the chemicals that cause migraine, depression, fatigue, skin and bowel disorders could be the cure.

Helen Franks
Prime Time £1.50

If you're a woman somewhere between your mid thirties and mid fifties, this is a book about you. 'Prime time' is the time when a woman has a chance to become truly herself, when the demands of being a wife and mother can take second place — a good time, but not all that easy. How do you pick up those pieces of yourself that didn't get a chance to blossom ten or twenty years ago? This compassionate, cogent and always honest look at the mid-life woman today covers such issues as sex, work, marriage, affairs, divorce, ageing and the menopause.

edited by Sigmund Stephen Miller
Symptoms – the complete home medical encyclopedia £2.50

The new medical encyclopedia – accurate, comprehensive, easy to use, sensible – enabling the reader to track down any symptom of ill health and identify, quickly and accurately, the causal disorder. *Symptoms* will tell you exactly what is wrong, and guide you in what action to take, whether a simple home remedy, or whether to seek advice from your doctor. Each section of the book is written by a specialist in one area of the body, and there is also a glossary of medical terms, comprehensive cross-indexes, and a guide to maintaining a high standard of general good health.

Barbara Griggs
The Home Herbal £1.95

a handbook of simple remedies

As people increasingly turn to alternative medicines and therapies here is an authoritative and practical guide to herbal remedies for a whole range of minor medical problems and ailments where conventional medicine may fail to provide relief or produce unpleasant side-effects. The book is organized alphabetically under the medical problems from acne to whooping cough, suggesting herbal remedies, where to get them and how to use them. Additional chapters cover the preparation of medicines, where to find your herbs, stocks of herbs for family needs, common and Latin botanical names.

Dr Vernon Coleman
The Home Pharmacy £1.75

the consumer's guide to over-the-counter medication

Here at last is an easy-to-understand and practical guide to the enormous variety of medicines and brands on the chemist's shelf, with advice on ingredients, prices, and dangers to be avoided. In two parts, this book examines the manufacture and marketing of home medicines, medication and the law, home alternatives, drugs and your body. The main section suggests which medicines you should choose for each ailment, and the cause of each ailment. No health-conscious family should be without this guide.

Fiction

☐	**Options**	Freda Bright	£1.50p
☐	**The Thirty-nine Steps**	John Buchan	£1.50p
☐	**Secret of Blackoaks**	Ashley Carter	£1.50p
☐	**Hercule Poirot's Christmas**	Agatha Christie	£1.50p
☐	**Dupe**	Liza Cody	£1.25p
☐	**Lovers and Gamblers**	Jackie Collins	£2.50p
☐	**Sphinx**	Robin Cook	£1.25p
☐	**Ragtime**	E. L. Doctorow	£1.50p
☐	**My Cousin Rachel**	Daphne du Maurier	£1.95p
☐	**Mr American**	George Macdonald Fraser	£2.25p
☐	**The Moneychangers**	Arthur Hailey	£2.50p
☐	**Secrets**	Unity Hall	£1.75p
☐	**Black Sheep**	Georgette Heyer	£1.75p
☐	**The Eagle Has Landed**	Jack Higgins	£1.95p
☐	**Sins of the Fathers**	Susan Howatch	£3.50p
☐	**The Master Sniper**	Stephen Hunter	£1.50p
☐	**Smiley's People**	John le Carré	£1.95p
☐	**To Kill a Mockingbird**	Harper Lee	£1.95p
☐	**Ghosts**	Ed McBain	£1.75p
☐	**Gone with the Wind**	Margaret Mitchell	£3.50p
☐	**Blood Oath**	David Morrell	£1.75p
☐	**Platinum Logic**	Tony Parsons	£1.75p
☐	**Wilt**	Tom Sharpe	£1.75p
☐	**Rage of Angels**	Sidney Sheldon	£1.95p
☐	**The Unborn**	David Shobin	£1.50p
☐	**A Town Like Alice**	Nevile Shute	£1.75p
☐	**A Falcon Flies**	Wilbur Smith	£2.50p
☐	**The Deep Well at Noon**	Jessica Stirling	£2.50p
☐	**The Ironmaster**	Jean Stubbs	£1.75p
☐	**The Music Makers**	E. V. Thompson	£1.95p

Non-fiction

☐	**Extraterrestrial Civilizations**	Isaac Asimov	£1.50p
☐	**Pregnancy**	Gordon Bourne	£3.50p
☐	**Jogging From Memory**	Rob Buckman	£1.25p
☐	**The 35mm Photographer's Handbook**	Julian Calder and John Garrett	£5.95p
☐	**Travellers' Britain** }	Arthur Eperon	£2.95p
☐	**Travellers' Italy**		£2.50p
☐	**The Complete Calorie Counter**	Eileen Fowler	80p

☐	**The Diary of Anne Frank**	Anne Frank	£1.75p
☐	**And the Walls Came Tumbling Down**	Jack Fishman	£1.95p
☐	**Linda Goodman's Sun Signs**	Linda Goodman	£2.50p
☐	**Dead Funny**	Fritz Spiegl	£1.50p
☐	**How to be a Gifted Parent**	David Lewis	£1.95p
☐	**Victoria RI**	Elizabeth Longford	£4.95p
☐	**Symptoms**	Sigmund Stephen Miller	£2.50p
☐	**Book of Worries**	Robert Morley	£1.50p
☐	**Airport International**	Brian Moynahan	£1.75p
☐	**The Alternative Holiday Catalogue**	edited by Harriet Peacock	£1.95p
☐	**The Pan Book of Card Games**	Hubert Phillips	£1.75p
☐	**Food for All the Family**	Magnus Pyke	£1.50p
☐	**Just Off for the Weekend**	John Slater	£2.50p
☐	**An Unfinished History of the World**	Hugh Thomas	£3.95p
☐	**The Baby and Child Book**	Penny and Andrew Stanway	£4.95p
☐	**The Third Wave**	Alvin Toffler	£2.75p
☐	**Pauper's Paris**	Miles Turner	£2.50p
☐	**The Flier's Handbook**		£5.95p

All these books are available at your local bookshop or newsagent, or can be ordered direct from the publisher. Indicate the number of copies required and fill in the form below

10

....

Name_____
(Block letters please)

Address_____

_____

Send to CS Department, Pan Books Ltd, PO Box 40, Basingstoke, Hants
Please enclose remittance to the value of the cover price plus:
35p for the first book plus 15p per copy for each additional book ordered
to a maximum charge of £1.25 to cover postage and packing
Applicable only in the UK

While every effort is made to keep prices low, it is sometimes
necessary to increase prices at short notice. Pan Books reserve
the right to show on covers and charge new retail prices which
may differ from those advertised in the text or elsewhere